Chair Yoga for Seniors

A Stretching Handbook of Chair Yoga Exercises and
Training You Can Do At Home To Build Agility,
Strength, and for Healthy Aging

By

Teri Wheeler

Disclaimer

This publication is designed to provide competent and reliable information regarding the subject matter covered. However, the views expressed in this publication are those of the author alone, and should not be taken as expert instruction or professional advice. The reader is responsible for his or her own actions.

The author hereby disclaims any responsibility or liability whatsoever that is incurred from the use or application of the contents of this publication by the purchaser or reader. The purchaser or reader is hereby responsible for his or her own actions.

Table of Contents

Introduction

To thrive as we age, we must modify our routines and way of life. Exercise can be more challenging if you have joint discomfort, sore muscles, weariness, or other typical age-related conditions. These issues can inadvertently force seniors to lead a sedentary or inactive lifestyle. Regular exercise is one of the best strategies for seniors to lead healthy lives. Fortunately, chair yoga is a simple and inexpensive form of exercise that offers excellent health benefits that the elderly can take advantage of even with limited mobility. Chair yoga is gentle on your joints, unlike high-impact exercises like jogging, weightlifting, and plyometrics, and can be a stepping stone to other types of exercise.

The advantages of chair yoga for senior citizens are enormous, and they include;

1. Soothing and stretching sore muscles

2. Minimizing chronic pain

3. Lowering stress levels

4. Enhancing circulation

5. Eases tension

6. Lowers blood pressure

7. Improves strength and balance

8. Promotes overall wellbeing

Now without further ado, let's journey through all you need to know to get started with chair yoga.

Chapter 1

Chair Yoga Basics

What is Chair Yoga?

Sitting or standing while holding onto the chair for support is a unique variation of yoga known as chair yoga.

When Lakshmi Voelker first developed chair yoga, it was intended for people with limited mobility, poor fitness levels, sight or balance impairments, and frailty. It has since become a therapeutic movement practice for people of all ages.

Yoga positions that may be performed seated or while holding a chair as a prop are commonly known as chair yoga poses.

When doing restorative yoga postures like Cat/Cow, which entails lying down on your hands and knees with your back flat on the mat, it is common to move through spinal flexion and extension while keeping your back horizontal at the same time.

A chair yoga version of this yoga posture is available for those unable to go down on their knees to practice yoga on the floor. In chair yoga, you can move to the front edge of the chair and perform the same two poses while flexing and extending your spine from a vertical position rather than from a horizontal one.

In a yoga studio, senior center, or rehabilitation institution, chair yoga may be taught in a group environment, or you can practice at home by following a video or conducting your own chair yoga poses.

Benefits of Chair Yoga

Although it's commonly known that regular exercise has several health benefits that continue far into old age, there is a risk when doing high-intensity workouts as your body becomes more fragile. There is a greater chance of discomfort and damage, and the rehabilitation process takes longer. You can tone up your entire body without putting yourself at risk of injury with chair yoga. When it comes to movement concerns such as arthritis and vertigo, chair yoga is ideal.

Let's take a closer look at the many advantages of chair yoga, using a chair as a prop.

1. Enhanced Adaptability

Yoga has long been known for its ability to improve flexibility, and chair yoga is no different. Chair yoga encourages the body to challenge itself by stretching it in unexpected places. As a result, the ability to perform daily duties becomes more efficient.

2. Enhances Muscle Power

Chair yoga is a great way to build and develop your muscles. Balance and mobility can be improved due to this, as well as the ability to bend. Gaining muscle also serves as a form of damage prevention for your body.

3. Balance and Coordination Can Be Improved

Through the transition of positions, chair yoga improves your body's spatial awareness. Yoga encourages you to use every part of your body to its fullest potential, allowing you to feel more in touch with your body and more aware of it. Eventually, you'll be able to develop your balance while also improving your coordination.

4. Inhibits Anxiety

Breathing and movement patterns are two aspects of yoga that aid concentration. This is a great way to alleviate some of the pressures of daily living. Yoga also requires you to meditate, which can help you relax and alleviate any stress you may be feeling.

5. Better Pain Management

When you exercise, a hormone called endorphins is released, which not only makes you feel better but also lessens your pain and suffering. You may also hear the term "natural painkillers" used to describe the effects of chair yoga, which teaches you to calm down and breathe through discomfort.

6. Improves the Quality of One's Sleep

Your body's sleep-wake cycle is better regulated when you exercise consistently. There are many benefits to chair yoga, including a low-intensity workout that doesn't exhaust the body.

7. Boosts Self-esteem and Alleviates Symptoms of Depression and Anxiety in Patients

Yoga, including chair yoga, has been shown in studies to help people of all ages reduce their symptoms of despair and anxiety. You'll feel rejuvenated and lighter after your yoga session because of the intense concentration required.

Who wouldn't want to begin practicing chair yoga after learning about its many advantages? It's good for the holy trinity of wellbeing: physical, mental, and emotional – and it's not too taxing on the body. Anyone of any age can benefit from this, so why wait?

Chair Yoga Mindset

Every area of your life is influenced by your mentality. The ideas you have about a person or issue can enhance your experience. They may also make it a terrible experience. When it comes to chair yoga, the same holds true. Adopt this mindset before you begin your practice on the mat (or in your chair) to get the most out of your time.

Also, how flexible your spine determines how healthy your body is.

There are three key functions that the spine performs:

1. Internal organs, as well as the spinal cord, are safeguarded
2. Keeping you upright and balanced; while

3. Allowing for a range of motion.

In order to achieve this, the spine is flexed in all directions in all types of yoga, including chair yoga. You bend forward, twist, backbend, and invert your body in a variety of ways. When you practice yoga in class, remember that you're doing so to improve your spine's overall health. This has a wide range of implications for your nervous and muscular systems, among other parts of your body.

In lieu of the above, let's see how you can adopt a good chair yoga mindset before exercising

1. Adopt a Beginner's Mind

The traditional origin of the term "beginner's mind" is the Zen meditation practice, and it refers to the state of mind when you are not trying to make something happen. You should avoid forcing a result or consequence.

This is particularly crucial when starting something new (like chair yoga). You want to approach the experience with an open mind and a sense of curiosity about how it will unfold. This will make practice more pleasurable. Additionally, it will enable you to acquire

13

the precise benefits you require in unexpected and exciting ways.

2. Observe Your Breathing

Just like you use metrics to measure the performance of your yoga business, you need a benchmark to track your development when practicing chair yoga. This benchmark is your breath.

In the majority of yoga classes, nasal breathing is utilized. This not only warms and moistens the air with each inhale and induces the relaxation response with each exhale but also allows you to gauge your level of exertion based on your breathing rate.

For instance, if you are in a lateral bend, as shown in the figure below, you are expending more energy to lift your arms and stretch to the side. If breathing becomes difficult and shallow, you have gone too far. You are exerting too much effort and must relax in the stance.

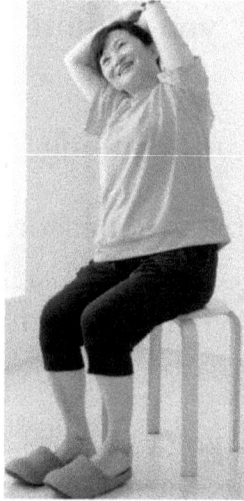

In chair yoga, you can focus on your breathing to determine when to push harder, when to take it easy, and when you've reached the optimal point when your breathing rate supports your movements.

3. Focus on Progression, Not Perfection

Due to the media's portrayal of yoga as an activity for persons already exceptionally flexible, many people neglect yoga as a useful training tool. You see the incredibly powerful in pretzel-like poses in advertisements and on social media. However, yoga is much more than the appearance of any specific posture.

In fact, when practicing chair yoga, you will likely not perform any of the moves seen in advertisements. Instead, you should concentrate on the physical progress you accomplish. You can answer questions like:

a) Where are you most powerful?
b) Are there existing areas of the body that are roomier or pain-free?
c) Can you take a deeper breath under hard yoga and life situations?

When you focus on the steps you're taking toward your goals rather than the vision of a flawless yoga pose, you'll be much more encouraged to continue your chair yoga practice.

Precautions for Safe Chair Yoga

Although Chair Yoga is a relatively accessible practice, basic safety considerations must be observed, as with any practice. Falls are the biggest cause of injury-related mortality in the elderly, and practitioners of this yoga type must feel as though they are firmly planted in their chairs as they would on a mat.

Before beginning a chair yoga exercise, ensure to review your health. Knee replacement surgery, osteoporosis, degenerative disk disease or other spinal disorders, hip replacements, heart attacks, and rotator cuff injuries are examples of health conditions that may prevent participation. Inner-ear issues or vertigo may also impede your ability to enjoy traditional yoga, but the seated variation is accessible. Before commencing, chairs should be placed on a nonslip surface, such as a yoga mat, and wheelchairs should be locked into place.

Although standard Yoga supports, such as blocks, are not typically utilized, straps may be used for some postures. A thorough warm-up is especially crucial because you may use muscles that are rarely used. Pay special attention to Yogic breathing; those with mobility challenges may not be accustomed to taking full, deep breaths, and the increase in oxygen will be of great benefit. People with cancer are not advised to hold their breath since they require the maximum amount of oxygen.

Some Chair Yoga participants choose to wear street clothes, which is acceptable so long as they are not confining. If feasible, shoes should be removed to allow the feet to flex.

According to a study conducted by California State University, one of the benefits of Chair Yoga is an increase in bone density. Additionally, Chair Yoga practitioners feel the same stress release and enhanced flexibility as traditional Yoga practitioners. Diabetics may experience enhanced blood flow to extremities, and the aerobic activity will strengthen the blood vessels of all yoga participants.

Chair Yoga may be a very beneficial complement to any Yogi's practice, and the message emphasizing ability rather than limitation should be taken to heart.

Among the general safety tips are the following:

- Inhale-Exhale. Inhaling and exhaling action relaxes the muscles and joints.

- Sit with your shoulders retracted from your ears and your head in alignment with your spine.

- Align the knee over the ankle to prevent excessive stress on the front of the knee. Keep your feet flat on the floor for stability.

- Avoid overexertion.

- Refrain from jerking or bouncing.

- Follow the chair yoga exercise as described in this book to improve your strength, flexibility and balance, and adhere to the duration of each pose. Yoga can be practiced every day. However, it is recommended that those who engage in severe activity must rest at least one day every week.

Chapter 2

Getting Started With Chair Yoga

What You Need To Start

It's a great idea to speak with your doctor before starting any new workout plan to receive a medical clearance and talk over any possible issues or adjustments that may be required, particularly if you're over 40 or have any pre-existing health concerns. Once you've been given the green light, you can begin your chair yoga exercise.

You will need the necessary equipment if you wish to practice chair yoga at home. The right chair will minimize your chance of injuries and help you get the most out of your activity. Use a sturdy, armless chair that won't rock, wobble, or wheel. Make sure your training area is level and flat such that the chair is aligned with the floor. An office chair on wheels or overstuffed armchairs is not appropriate for chair yoga. A chair that allows you to place both feet flat on the floor and naturally positions your hips slightly higher than your knees is highly recommended. To prevent slippage, place the chair on a solid surface such as a carpet or a yoga mat. You can also place the back of the chair against a wall for added stability. You would also need to wear comfortable and flexible clothing that would enable you to exercise well enough.

If you will be attending a chair yoga class, everything you need should be provided, along with the chair; therefore, all you need to take with you is comfortable clothing, slip-resistant shoes or socks, a water bottle to stay hydrated, and a towel should you perspire or need more cushioning.

Yoga props such as blocks, straps, and resistance bands that are commonly used in mat practices are not required for chair yoga unless you want to challenge yourself.

Best Time of Day To Exercise

To put it in the simplest words possible, the ideal time to practice yoga is whenever it is convenient for you. Given that the key to reaping all of yoga's numerous advantages is constant practice over the course of time (and hopefully for a very long time into the future), you will need to find a routine that is compatible with your way of life and is practical for your schedule. Because of the changes in your life, this might shift with time.

For several years, perhaps, you've been attending yoga lessons in the evening immediately after you get home from work. However, as you started a family, it became more practical for you to go very early in the morning before work or during the day when your children were at school. As long as you find a schedule that you can stick to, the actual times and days of the week you practice yoga doesn't really matter as much as finding a routine you can maintain. Instead of attempting to squeeze your yoga practice around the rest of your obligations, make room for it in your schedule.

Advantages of Practicing Yoga in the Morning

It is recommended in certain schools of yoga to perform yoga postures very early in the morning, if at all possible, before the sun rises. Beginning your day with a session of yoga can help you feel more energized and clear-headed, and it can also help set the stage for the remainder of your day. It is common for people to have morning routines that are easier to control or more predictable, which might make it simpler to maintain a consistent daily practice. In addition, many people discover that they have more strength and stamina for physical activity first thing in the morning, as opposed to the last thing at night after a long day. In order to prevent stomach cramps and indigestion, some people find it helpful to practice yoga on an empty stomach.

Activities that need you to use a lot of energy are not recommended first thing in the morning.

Advantages of Practicing Yoga in the Afternoon

You can help yourself de-stress after a hectic morning by doing some yoga in the afternoon before dinner. This will also help you work up an appetite for the next meal. If you would rather practice yoga in the middle of the day, you should wait at least two to three hours after eating before engaging in yoga.

In addition, the later in the day it is, the more warmed up your muscles are likely to be, as opposed to first thing in the morning, when you are likely to feel stiffer. In comparison to when your muscles feel tight, later in the day, when they have had more time to relax, you may be able to put in a bit more effort toward increasing your flexibility. It's possible that if you do yoga in the afternoon, you'll be able to have the best of both worlds. If this is when you have more energy, then a demanding and strenuous practice would be beneficial for you at this time. However, if you need to wind down toward the end of your workday, it may be more restorative for you to do so.

Advantages of Practicing Yoga in the Evening

Your nighttime yoga practice can help relieve stress and promote relaxation, which will allow you to decompress and enjoy the rest of your day. As a result, practicing yoga in the evening can be an effective component of a reassuring bedtime routine that can assist you in getting ready for sleep.

What To Do Before You Start Exercising

Having some water before starting your exercise routine and immediately after is a great idea. Most seniors are known to have little to or water, thus becoming subject to lots of dehydration. Additionally, it would be best if you didn't eat before starting your exercise routine, typically 1hr before you start. This will help you exercise more comfortably.

Setting Up Your Yoga Space

Building a sacred space for yoga at home is a wonderful act of self-respect. Having a designated area for your yoga and movement practice will help you make it a regular part of your life and emphasize the significance of your work.

Here are some suggestions for making your home conducive to practicing yoga.

First, locate a comfortable spot to position your chair. Having a specific location to practice at will encourage regularity. You'll be more likely to actually start practicing yoga if you don't have to waste mental energy deciding where to set up your chair. There is a common misconception that people can't do chair yoga at home because there isn't enough space. But you really don't need that much space to practice. Your chair and some floor space that is sufficient to stretch around are all that is required, most of the time. A lot of room isn't necessary. It's fine to use a room that serves multiple purposes as your "yoga studio" at home. A spare nook in the living room might do, as would the wall space right beside your bed. Even if you only have a little bit of space, you can still practice chair yoga.

Second, create an environment free of disruptions. Pick a location that has access to natural light and is quiet and undisrupted. Your designated yoga area should be a calm, undisturbed spot for you to stretch and relax. You can even do your training outside if you reside in a mild environment. In my last residence, I converted the garage into a personal yoga studio. Natural light and breezes were two of my favorite features. A quiet spot on a patio or balcony would work just as well as a designated Zen space.

The third step is to maintain a tidy and well-organized environment. You'll be more motivated to make use of your area if you take the time to keep it clean and organized. Get rid of the mess and put everything back where it belongs. Keeping your physical environment tidy might help you keep your mental environment tidy as well. I make an effort to store away everything I use, even if I plan to retrieve it all again the following day. Like making the bed, keeping my yoga workspace tidy is a habit for me, and it takes only one minute to do.

Embellishing the area is the fourth stage. Create an environment that you'll like spending time in. Even on the days when you'd rather stay in bed, this spot should motivate you to get out there and practice. Plants, a gorgeous tapestry, incense, or crystals are just a few examples of what you may use to transform your yoga area into a tranquil sanctuary. Maybe you like a bare, minimalist room without any decorative accents.

To sum up, I would encourage you to set up your yoga space in front of a mirror where you can get instantaneous feedback on how well you are executing the poses; not so important, though, but really helpful, if you can.

A Short message from the Author:

Hey, I hope you are enjoying the book? I would love to hear your thoughts!

Many readers do not know how hard reviews are to come by and how much they help an author.

Customer Reviews

★★★★★ 2

5.0 out of 5 stars ▾

5 star		100%
4 star		0%
3 star		0%
2 star		0%
1 star		0%

See all verified purchase reviews ›

Share your thoughts with other customers

Write a customer review

I would be incredibly grateful if you could take just 60 seconds to write a short review on Amazon, even if it is a few sentences!

>> Click here to leave a quick review

Thanks for the time taken to share your thoughts!

Chapter 3

Warming Up Poses

Warm-ups are essential when practicing chair yoga. If you've ever arrived early to a yoga class, you might have seen your fellow students warming up with some simple poses. It's true that you can get warmed up for yoga by practicing various yoga postures. The flexibility and muscular tone you gain from these stretches will serve you well during your workout.

Warming up before any physical activity helps to avoid injury and improves performance. Warm-ups for chair yoga take a few minutes, so don't neglect them. Blood flow to muscles rises by up to 75% after only five to ten minutes of warm-up activities. It is customary in yoga to begin with warm-ups, such as sun salutations. Greeting the sun by moving the body with the breath helps put us in the right mental state to flow and move more easily.

Warm-up flows can be thought of as movement meditations. We frequently go about our days aimlessly. When we take the time to connect our breath to our activity, our mind and body become more connected, and we have a clearer perspective on our day. We also begin to live with more purpose and clarity. It's incredible to believe that a few conscious motions can have such an impact, but they can! Warming up can be done as slowly or quickly as you wish. Each time you execute the workout, your pace may vary. Pay attention to your body and your breath, and be sure to connect the two as you move. Your breathing and movement should be coordinated. Make sure there are no distractions. Before you begin your practice, turn off or silence your computer and phone. Remember that chair yoga warm-ups are similar to mat warm-ups in a conventional yoga class. The main difference is that chair yoga warm-ups are done while seated in a chair!

Importance of Warming Up

A proper warm-up has several advantages. The risk of harm is diminished to begin with. If you jump directly into complex yoga poses without warming up, you risk injuring yourself and taking some time off from exercising.

Preparing your body for yoga by warming up is essential. To buttress what has been highlighted earlier, warm-up is helpful for your muscles since it elevates your body temperature. This makes them more flexible and open to the positive effects of yoga. Skipping a warm-up makes it more difficult to keep good posture throughout the day. To get the most out of yoga, you need to have good posture, and if you don't, you risk injuring your muscles, tendons, and joints. Besides, warming up with some stretches is a terrific way to feel better during your workout. Once you've gotten into the swing of things with your routine, you'll be prepared for whatever comes your way.

Below is a variety of effective chair yoga warm-up poses that you can use to get your yoga practice started off on the right foot.

So, if you're ready, then let's get started!

Sun Salutation Arm

A seated sun salutation is a fantastic alternative whether you're practicing chair yoga due to physical limitations, mobility concerns, or simply the desire for a break while seated at your computer. With this type of pose, the spine is lengthened, and the tension in the shoulders and neck is released.

1. Sitting tall, take a deep breath in and bring your arms up, palms facing up.
2. Exhale and float your arms back down to your sides.
3. Repeat 5 times more.

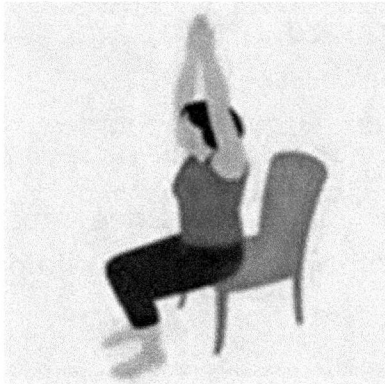

Mountain Pose

One of the fundamental grounding postures in yoga is the mountain pose, which is frequently employed as a transitional or relaxing pose between other poses. This pose helps you to contract your core, engage your posture, and establish a connection with your breathing.

1. Place your ears over your shoulders and your shoulders over your hips as you sit tall in your chair.
2. Position your feet on the floor so that they are hip-width apart.
3. Position your sitting bones so that they are evenly distributed on the chair.
4. Lightly contract your abdominal muscles and bring your navel in toward your spine and slightly upward.
5. Open your chest.
6. Roll your shoulder blades backward and downward.
7. Place your hands on either your thighs or your knees for support. The mountain posture can be seen here.

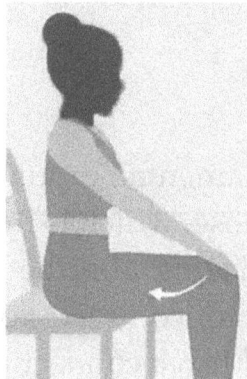

8. Now, place one hand on your abdominal region and the other hand, on your chest, directly over your heart.
9. If doing so does not cause you any discomfort, you should start breathing in and out via your nose. It is important to make deliberate use of your diaphragm, as it is your body's major muscle responsible for respiration.
10. When you inhale, draw your diaphragm down toward your abdomen and allow your abdomen to rise.
11. During the exhale, you should relax your diaphragm and allow your abdomen to relax.
12. Your hand on your stomach should go up and down in rhythm with your breathing.
13. Maintain this breathing for five to ten complete breath cycles.

Cat-Cow

The intention of this pose is to stretch and extend the spine. The posture's "cat" portion folds the spine forward. The cow is a soft backbend that helps in opening the heart of the shoulders and its front.

1. Sit in the "mountain pose" position, with your hands placed on your thighs.
2. As you inhale, arch your back and see whether you can glance up without straining your neck.

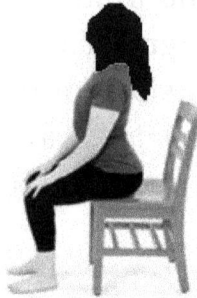

3. Your shoulders should be rolled downward and away from your ears.
4. While you are exhaling, circle the small of your back, draw your navel in toward your spine, and glance at your navel. This is a sitting version of the cat pose.

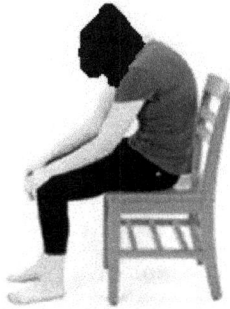

5. Continue this sequence 35 times

Side Stretch

Stretching is good for seniors because it increases awareness and encourages full use of the diaphragm.

1. Seated in the mountain pose, take a deep breath in and raise your right arm aloft with your palm facing inside and your fingers pointing upward.
2. For added stability, you should rest your left hand on the chair seat.

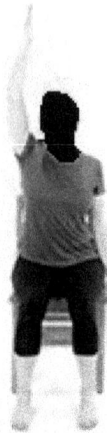

3. Let your breath out gradually and tilt your body to the left. Maintain a very small bend in both of your elbows.

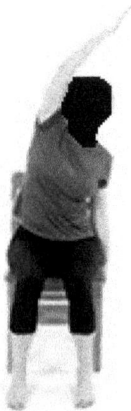

4. Take a deep breath in and come back to the center.
5. Let your breath out and bring your right arm down.
6. Repeat the same sequence on the opposite side.

Seated Twist

Twisting poses are beneficial because they alleviate lower back discomfort, improve digestion, and boost circulation. These poses are frequently referred to as "detox" poses. Even if your chair has a back, you shouldn't make use of it to draw yourself farther into the twist. Keep this in mind at all times. Do not try to force your body past its natural stopping point by pulling too hard. Your body will find its own stopping point. Forced twists can result in catastrophic injury.

1. You should be seated in the mountain pose
2. Extend your spine even more as you take a breath in and raise your arms up and out to the sides of your body as you do so.
3. Exhale, and while you're doing so, slowly rotate your upper body to the right. From this position, your left hand will rest by your side, and your

right hand will rest on the back of the chair, assisting you as you twist calmly.

4. Take a quick glance to your right over your shoulder. Maintain the twist with the support of your grasp on the chair, but do not allow it to get more severe.

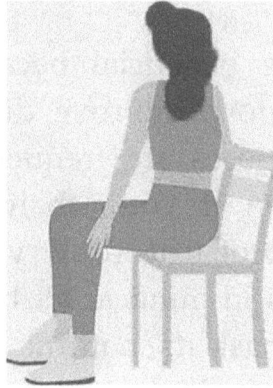

5. After five deep breaths, return to the starting position (the front) and repeat the twist on your body's left side.

Note: Take special care to avoid twisting so much, especially if you suffer from osteoporosis or lower back pain. Your arms should be kept downward at your sides if it makes you feel any better. To avoid straining your lower back, ensure not to pull further into the twist with your hands and arms.

Neck Stretch

You can restore your flexibility and range of motion with neck stretches. You may go about your everyday business easily because of it.

1. Sit in the "mountain pose" position.
2. Lengthen your spine as you inhale, working from your sitting bones all the way up to the crown of your head.

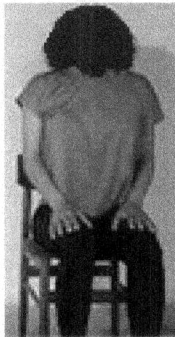

3. Exhale, and as you're doing so, slowly move your head forward. Your chin should be directed toward your chest.

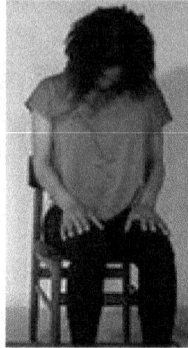

4. Take a deep breath in and look upward while jutting out your chin. As you exhale, move your chin closer to your chest.

5. Keep at this movement for a few breaths (inhalations and exhalations).

6. During your inhale, bring your head into a neutral position. While you are exhaling, turn your head to the right and move your nose to that side. Inhale, then bring your attention back to the center. Exhale, then turn your head to the left as you shift your nose to the left.

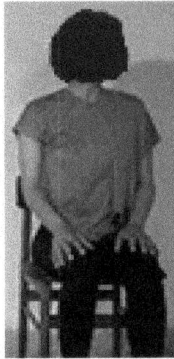

Nose to the left   Nose to the right

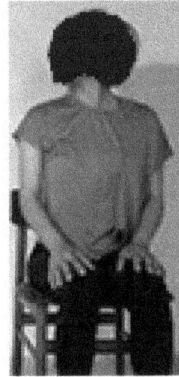

Here is another method you can try out

1. Seated in a mountain pose, place your right hand across your head. Then, grab a tiny patch of your head's left side.
2. Gradually and gently nudge your right ear some centimeters nearer to your right shoulder.
3. Keep your shoulders in a relaxed and comfortable spot, breathing normally. Only stretch if it seems comfortable for you; don't compel yourself to do so. Try to imagine how stretching feels for you.

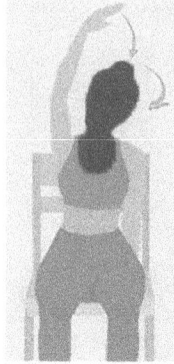

4. On the subsequent exhalation, return to the seated mountain pose position.
5. Your left hand should hold onto your head's right side.
6. Bring your left ear all the way over to your left shoulder.

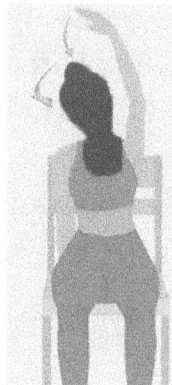

7. Compare the degree of the stretch between this side and the opposite side.
8. Sit comfortably in the mountain pose position on your subsequent exhalation.

Forward Fold

The complete back line of the body is lengthened in this sitting variation of a forward fold. Additionally, it serves as a resting position and a means to focus inward. Releasing strain in the hips, neck, lower back, or shoulders is facilitated by the seated forward fold.

1. Deepen your breathing as your legs are folded in the seated mountain position while concentrating on lengthening your spine.

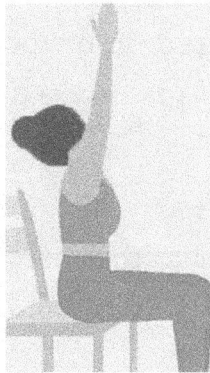

Position your hands on your thighs to support yourself while folding or keeping them by your sides.

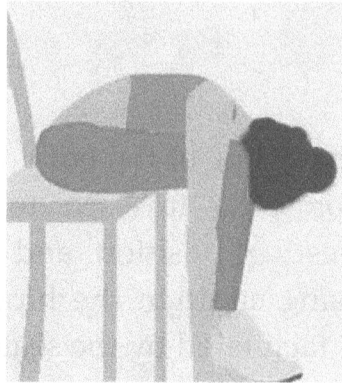

2. This pose stretches your back muscles while gently lengthening your spine, which supports digestion. In this pose, evenly breathe five or more spaced breaths.
3. When prepared, your torso should be raised back to an upright posture while breathing in.

Half Forward Fold

This pose is similar to the forward fold, except that you would be making a 45-degree "half" fold.

1. Seated in a mountain pose, take a deep breath in and raise your arms aloft with your palms facing inside and your fingers pointing upward.

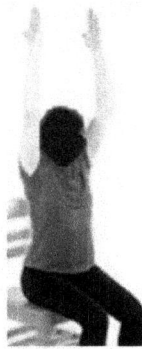

2. Let your breath out as you bend forward from the hips to create a 45-degree angle with your body and thighs.

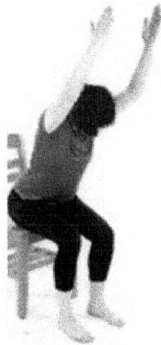

3. Keep your head in line with your spine and your back straight at all times.
4. Hold for three to five breaths.
5. Take a breath in and bring your torso back to an upright position.
6. Let your breath out and bring your arms to your sides.

Chapter 4

Strength, Balance, and Flexibility Poses

Muscle mass and metabolism declines with age, and seniors who lead sedentary lives frequently suffer from maintaining their balance. Seniors who maintain an active lifestyle and engage in balance training are often better able to respond to the demands of everyday life and are better able to prevent falling.

The Centers for Disease Control and Prevention (CDCP) report that one-third of American adults over the age of 65 will have a fall at some point during the year. Because falls are the second greatest cause of brain and spinal cord injuries in older adults, balance training is very crucial during this stage of life. Falls are the major cause of damage to the spinal cord. Therefore, it is essential for older individuals to maintain their balance and flexibility in order to sustain their health and general wellbeing. By doing so, they can lower their risk of injury and maintain their mobility as they age. This is crucial because 3 million older persons visit the emergency room each year after suffering injuries from falls. In a 2010 study, seniors in a retirement home engaged in twice-weekly yoga sessions for a period of 12 weeks. The majority of poses were performed while seated or standing with a chair used for balance. Participants exhibited improved lower-body flexibility and static balance at the conclusion of the trial. Additionally, they were less afraid of falling and felt more confident in their physical prowess.

People who are unable to attend traditional yoga classes can still engage in workout sessions to train their balance, strength, and flexibility by engaging in chair yoga exercises. Chair yoga is an efficient approach to train for balance, strength, and flexibility. The most effective aspects of flexibility and balance training are combined in chair yoga poses.

The following chair yoga sequence aims to improve your ability to perform activities of daily living. Maintaining each pose for about a minute and a half is recommended.

Downward Facing Dog

In a lot of chair yoga lessons, this downward dog version is typical. By varying how far back and how far forward you fold, you may change the level of intensity.

In either case, you will lengthen the sides of your body and hamstrings whilst still strengthening your arms, core, and hip stabilizing muscles.

1. Take a position in front of your chair. You can position the chair so that either the front or the back is facing you, depending on which provides a more comfortable working height for you.
2. Put your hands on the chair, and while doing so, walk your feet back until your back is in a straight position. Your feet are planted at a distance equal to the breadth of your hips.
3. Put some pressure on the chair with your hands. Bring your shoulder blades together and down your back. Open your chest. Put some upward pressure on your sitting bones. Put your entire back and shoulders through some stretches. Take a breath here. Please remain still for a few deep breaths (about 5-10 breaths.

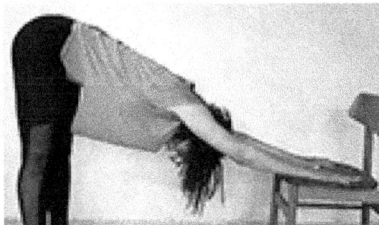

Boat Pose

One of the top chair yoga poses for core strength is the boat pose. It calls for the use of numerous distinct muscles in the abdomen, combining balance with strength via the legs. You have the option of performing this pose with either one leg at a time or both legs at the same time.

1. Take a seat on the chair with the back of your sitting bones facing the chair's edge. Check that you are still experiencing a sense of ease and stability. From this vantage point, you can elevate either one of your legs or both of them. Put your hands behind your knees and grab hold of the backs of your thighs. Activate your core. Your navel should also be pulled in and up.

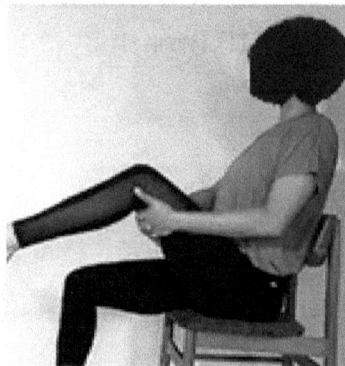

2. Establish your balanced position. You are free to try out a few things in this position if you choose. Make an effort to release your grip on your legs and stretch your arms out in front of you. You might also provide your best effort to straighten your legs while maintaining your grip on the backs of your thighs. This is an excellent pose for working on one's core. Don't forget to take deep breaths of about 3-5.

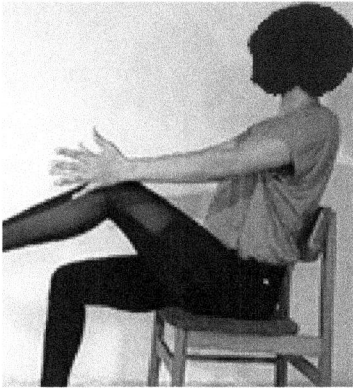

Eagle Pose

The eagle pose enhances posture and provides more awareness for the body as well as balance and concentration. With this pose, your thighs are strengthened, including your ankles, core, and legs, while also stretching your upper back, thighs, and shoulders.

1. Sit in the mountain pose position. Put your left leg over your right one and then cross your legs. You can put your right foot behind your left leg if you have the space to do so. Your legs should be intertwined. Your upper arms should be crossed, with your right arm on top.
2. Give yourself a shoulder massage by putting your hands on your shoulders and giving yourself a hug. Bring the palms of your hands together in this position. You might also tie your lower arms together and bring your hands together instead. No matter what you do, bring your elbows up to your sides.

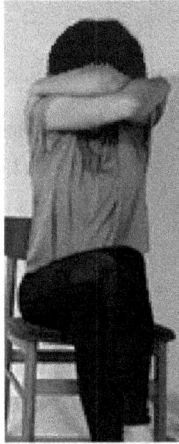

3. Put some pressure on your forearms and turn them so that they are facing away from your face. While working on strengthening your core and shoulders, you will also receive a great stretch in your glutes and rhomboids. Always keep your core engaged, and don't forget to breathe. Hold this position for a few more breaths (about 5 or more).

High Lunge Pose

This pose is very useful if you are unable to bend your back leg's toes in a high lunge pose.

1. Turn your torso to the right as you bring your right leg and foot closer to the right side of the chair. Grab the chair for support and stability. Put your left leg in a straight position behind you. Make a coiled motion with your left foot's toes. Check that the front of your right knee is positioned above your ankle. Find your balanced position and engage your core muscles.
2. You have the choice to extend your arms upward toward the heavens. You can also reach the left arm upward while retaining your grip with the right hand on the back of the chair. Your hip flexor will feel a nice stretch after holding this pose.

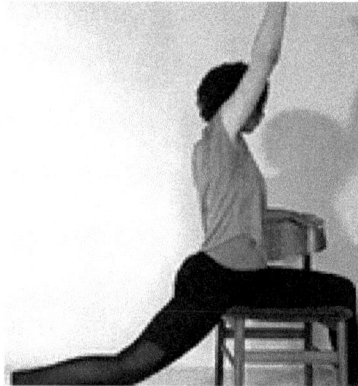

3. Take a short break here to catch your breath, and then repeat the process on the other side.

Note: You can position a block underneath your front foot.

Reverse Arm Hold

This pose will cause an opening of your chest and the stretching of your shoulders, thereby helping with stress, posture, and breathing challenges.

1. Stretch your arms wide and inhale while keeping your palms down.

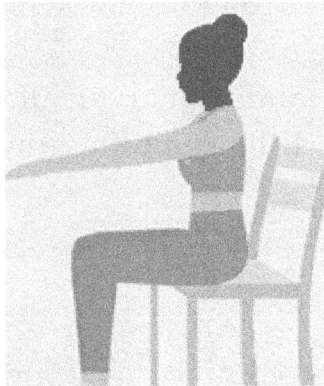

2. Swing your arms beyond your back, flex your elbows, and exhale by rolling your shoulders slightly forward such that your palms are facing behind you.

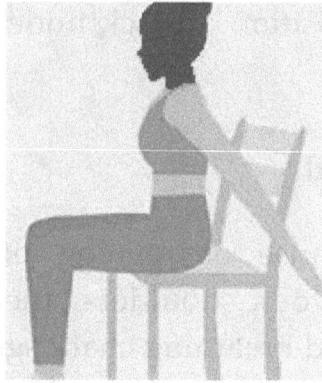

3. Clasp your hands together (elbows, fingers, wrists, hands), in a manner that's convenient then gradually pull them apart without letting go of the grip.
4. After five calm, equal breaths with the arms clasped, hold the opposite arm in place for five breaths.

Camel Pose

The backbend stretch known as "Camel Pose" stretches the entire front of the body. This pose can be a fantastic method to ease back and neck pain brought on by hunching over a computer or when driving.

In detail, this pose;

- Stretches the whole body's front, throat, chest, thighs, abdomen, and groins.
- Bolsters the back muscles
- Enhances posture
- Boosts the stomach and neck organs

1. Take a seat on the chair with the back of your sitting bones facing the chair's edge. Check that you are still experiencing a sense of ease and stability pushed through with the soles of both feet.
2. Now, lay the palms of your hands on the small of your back with your fingers pointing downward. To improve your posture, roll your shoulder blades down and backward. Open your chest. You should only gaze up if it doesn't put too much strain on your neck.

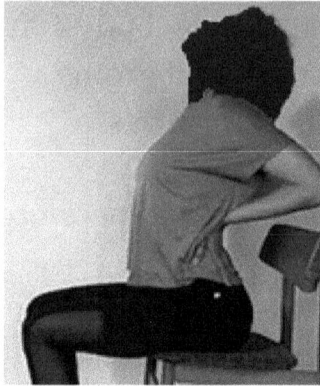

3. Take some slow, deep breaths right now.

Note: You can grip onto the outer corners of your chair if you are unable to reach your lower back.

Warrior II Pose

This will stretch every muscle in your body by activating your upper body, lower body, and core. The goal of Warrior Pose II is to promote balance and self-assurance. Even though this position is powerful when performed standing, the advantages gained here are more in the direction of balance and strength.

1. Maintain good posture by sitting on the edge of your seat.

2. While pressing your outer heel down, bend your right knee to the side and stretch your left leg out behind you. Your right knee should remain bent.

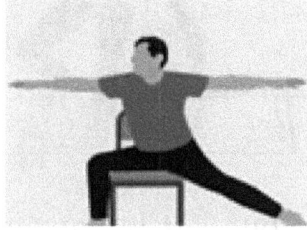

3. After holding this position for five breaths, switch sides and continue the exercise.

Tree Pose

Activating the standing foot in the tree pose aids in finding balance and stability.

1. Standing with the chair on your right side, face the back of the chair.
2. Put your right hand on the chair.

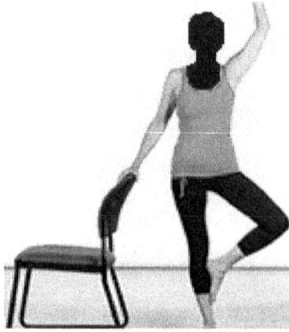

3. By rotating your left leg away from your body, position your heel above your ankle or your whole foot on the calf muscle.
4. Raise your left arm above your head and breathe for some breathing cycles.
5. Repeat with the other leg.

The end... almost!

Hey! We've made it to the final chapter of this book, and I hope you've enjoyed it so far.

If you have not done so yet, I would be incredibly thankful if you could take just a minute to leave a quick review on Amazon

Reviews are not easy to come by, and as an independent author with a little marketing budget, I rely on you, my readers, to leave a short review on Amazon.

Even if it is just a sentence or two!

So if you really enjoyed this book, please...

>> Click here to leave a brief review on Amazon.

I truly appreciate your effort to leave your review, as it truly makes a huge difference.

Chapter 5

Cool Down Poses

The poses used during the cool-down are just as vital as the more active exercises. Feeling the impact of the stretches, finding one's center, and relaxing are only some of the mental benefits gained from cool-down poses.

An effective cool down is a crucial aspect of any post-workout regimen. Though it may not aid in the alleviation of muscle discomfort, it is helpful in restoring the body to a balanced state post-workout activity. It's crucial to bring the body's temperature to a reduced level, to breathe more slowly, and return the heart rate to a normal range after your yoga activity is completed for the day. Yoga or no yoga, though, the body will naturally cool down. Yoga, however, can assist with the procedure, and it also has a number of other advantages that could prove useful as you approach the completion of your workout.

Try incorporating these yoga poses into your post-workout cool-down regimen.

Pigeon Pose

This seated variation of the pigeon pose does the same thing by stretching and strengthening the hips.

1. Take a seat on the chair with the back of your sitting bones facing the chair's edge. Check that you are still experiencing a sense of ease and stability.
2. Put your right ankle on top of the left knee or thigh, whichever is lower.
3. Breathe in for some breathing cycles and while breathing in, try to stretch your spine.
4. While exhaling, move your chest in the direction of your legs.

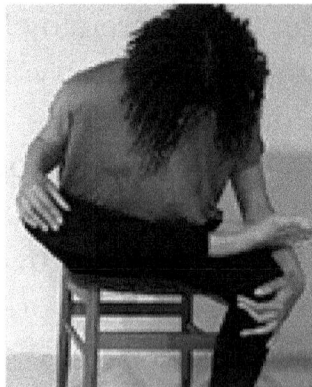

5. Hold this position and take a few deep breaths before moving on. Your glutes and lower back will benefit from this stretch.

6. To release yourself from the pose, take a deep breath in and lift your upper body up.

7. Exhale, and put your right foot back on the ground as you return to the starting position and repeat on the other side.

Note: If you are unable to position your foot on the opposite knee or thigh, you can try this alternative; On the inner part of the foot that is grounded, position a block or stack of blocks and then place your foot on top of it.

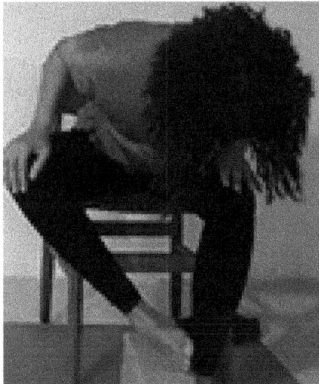

Child's Pose

The goal of the child's pose is to calm the mind and the body. Your thighs, spine, hips, and ankles are all stretched as a result. Additionally, it can reduce stress in your lower back muscles, hamstrings, chest, and shoulders.

You might need two chairs and a blanket in order to achieve this pose.

1. Take a seat in one of the chairs, and position the second chair in front of you, perhaps covering the seat with a blanket.
2. Inhale and stretch your spine. After letting out an exhale, position your head so that it is either between your legs or on the chair (covered by the blanket) in front of you.
3. Put the palms of your hands down on the chair in front of you with the fingers pointing down, or let your fingertips reach the floor in front of you.

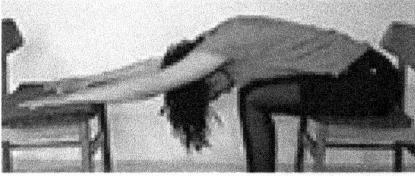

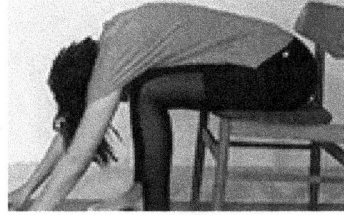

4. Take a few deep breaths. Stay for as long as you feel it's necessary or appropriate.

Hamstring Stretch

This pose stretches the hamstrings and calves while also engaging the core muscles, which enhances balance.

1. Beginning with the mountain pose, move forward until you are seated close to the chair's front edge.
2. While maintaining a bent knee on your left side and your foot planted firmly on the ground with your left foot, stretch your right leg in front of you. Put the back of your right heel on the ground, flex your right foot, and point the toes of your right foot up toward the ceiling.
3. Position both hands on the left side of your thigh and lean forward from the hips just a little bit. Always remember to prioritize your head over your heart.

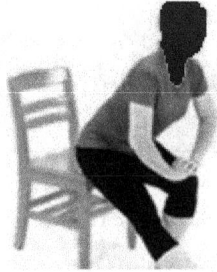

4. Hold for three to five breaths.
5. Perform the same steps on the other side.

Note: To prevent undue strain on the knee, you should steer clear of putting your hands on the straight leg.

You can put a strap or a cloth around the ball of your right foot and then elevate your right leg to give yourself a more severe stretch.

Corpse Pose

Corpse pose is a rehabilitative pose, and because it is therapeutic, it is used in treating lower back problems such as pain, inflammation, and spine rigidity. The fact that the intervertebral disc pressure greatly decreases when we lie on our backs is one of the chief reasons to use this pose in your everyday routine. Gravity drags us down since the majority of us spend much of the day in an upright position, either standing or sitting at a computer for extended periods of time.

This position balances the sympathetic and parasympathetic nervous systems by calming the nervous system to a significant degree. The body goes into a state of relaxation, which aids in healing.

Also, this pose will ease you into the rest of your day, helping your body to fully benefit from all the poses you've performed. You may choose to complete the exercise routine in the seated mountain pose.

1. Take a few deep breaths while seated.

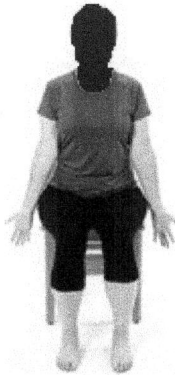

2. Focus your awareness on each aspect of your body. To feel more invigorated, you can try

working your way up from your feet to the top of your head. Alternately, you can begin from the top of your head and work your way down to your feet in order to achieve a more grounded sensation.

3. Revert to your regular daily activities whenever you feel ready to do so upon completion of this pose.

Conclusion

Because chair yoga poses allow you to avoid standing for too long unsupported, it is a good option for seniors with limited mobility. In addition to being beneficial for the elderly, these poses are also quite helpful for those who spend their days sitting at a desk for long and even those recovering from some muscular pain, among many others. Going to a yoga studio to engage in this stretching activity isn't all too necessary so long you have the resources and guidance for conducting these exercises in the comfort of your home, which is what this book helps you achieve. Keep in mind that if you have any health concerns, kindly check in with your doctor before practicing any poses discussed in the pages of this book.

So I urge you to bring your best YOU forward to ensure that you master these poses to build strength, balance, and flexibility while observing every safety precaution highlighted.

I wish you all the best!

www.ingramcontent.com/pod-product-compliance
Lightning Source LLC
Chambersburg PA
CBHW070029030426
42335CB00017B/2359